BODY WORKS™

BLOOD
The Circulatory System

Gillian Houghton

PowerKiDS press.

New York

Published in 2007 by The Rosen Publishing Group, Inc.
29 East 21st Street, New York, NY 10010

First Edition

Editor: Amelie von Zumbusch
Book Design: Greg Tucker

Photo Credits: Photo Credits: Cover © 3D4Medical.com/Getty Images; pp. 5, 14 (right) © J. Bavosi/Photo Researchers, Inc.; p. 6 © F. Leroy, Biocosmos/Photo Researchers; p. 9 (left) © Eaton/Custom Medical Stock Photo; pp. 9 (right), 14 (left), 17 (right) © Eye of Science/Photo Researchers, Inc.; p. 10 (left) © Zephyr/Photo Researchers, Inc.; p. 10 (right) © John W. Karapelou, CMI/Phototake; p. 13 (left) © Will & Deni McIntyre/Corbis; p. 13 (right) © Susumu Nishinaga/Photo Researchers, Inc.; p. 17 (left) © Biology Media/Photo Researchers, Inc; p. 18 (left) © SPL/Photo Researchers, Inc; p. 18 (right) © LADA/Photo Researchers, Inc.; p. 21 (left) © James Cavallini/Photo Researchers, Inc.; p. 21 (right) © Jens Nieth/zefa/Corbis.

Library of Congress Cataloging-in-Publication Data

Houghton, Gillian.
  Blood : the circulatory system / Gillian Houghton.— 1st ed.
     p. cm. — (Body works)
  Includes index.
  ISBN (10) 1-4042-3472-1 (13) 978-1-4042-3472-7 (library binding) — ISBN (10) 1-4042-2181-6 (13) 978-1-4042-2181-9 (pbk.)
  1. Cardiovascular system—Juvenile literature. I. Title. II. Series.
  QP103.H68 2007
  612.1—dc22
                                          2005035718

Manufactured in the United States of America

Contents

The Circulatory System

Your body is made up of many tiny parts called cells. All these cells need **nutrients** and **oxygen** to live and to work. Blood brings nutrients from the **digestive system** and oxygen from the **respiratory system** to the cells. As they work cells make waste, such as the gas carbon dioxide. This **harmful** gas is carried away from the cells by the blood.

Blood travels through the web of the circulatory system. The circulatory system is made up of the heart, the **blood vessels**, and the blood.

This is a drawing of the circulatory system. If you laid out all the blood vessels in your body in a straight line, it would be almost 60,000 miles (100,000 km) long.

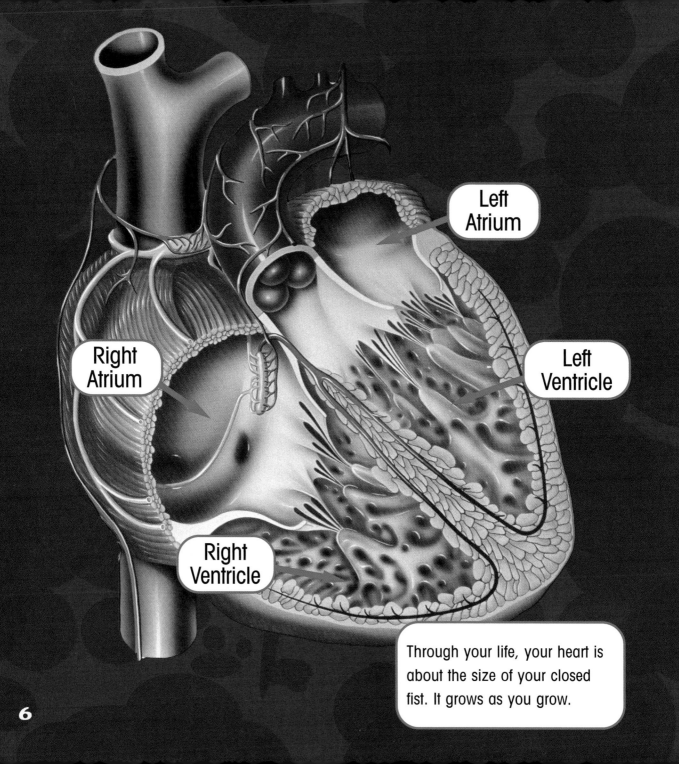

Left
Atrium

Right
Atrium

Left
Ventricle

Right
Ventricle

Through your life, your heart is
about the size of your closed
fist. It grows as you grow.

The Heart

The heart is an **organ** that lies between the **lungs**. It has four chambers, or parts. These chambers are called the right atrium, the right ventricle, the left atrium, and the left ventricle. Four valves form the walls between the chambers. The valves are made of **muscle** and strong ropes of **tissue** called tendons.

The heart powers the circulatory system. The heart's muscles press together about once every second when the body is at rest. This pumps, or pushes, blood through the heart's chambers and into the blood vessels.

The Blood Vessels

Blood vessels are tunnels of muscle that lead toward and away from the heart. Blood moves through the blood vessels. It goes to the parts of the body where it is needed. Then the blood returns to the heart.

There are three kinds of blood vessels. They are arteries, capillaries, and veins. Arteries carry blood away from the heart and toward the lungs and other parts of the body. Within organs and other tissues, arteries branch off into smaller vessels called capillaries. Veins carry blood from throughout the body back to the heart.

Veins

Arteries

The capillary above is carrying blood to the muscles. This capillary is shown at 6,900 times larger than its real size.

Air moves through the lungs into small tunnels called alveoli. The alveoli pass oxygen to the blood in the capillaries. *Inset:* This picture shows the arteries in the pulmonary circuit.

Blood and Oxygen

The circulatory system is made up of two circuits, or paths. The systemic circuit is made up of the blood vessels that bring oxygen to the cells and carry waste away from the cells.

The pulmonary circuit ties the circulatory system to the respiratory system. The heart pumps the oxygen-poor blood to the lungs. In the lungs the blood takes in a new supply of oxygen and gets rid of carbon dioxide. Then the oxygen-rich blood returns to the heart to be pumped through the systemic circuit.

Moving Nutrients

The circulatory system is tied to all the body's systems. For example, it is closely tied to the digestive system. The organs of the digestive system break down the food a person eats into nutrients. These nutrients move through the walls of the digestive organs and into the blood. The blood carries the nutrients to cells throughout the body. These cells use the nutrients to make energy. Energy is power to work or to act. Without the circulatory system, none of the body's cells could get the nutrients they need.

Your body gets the nutrients it needs from the food you eat. *Inset:* Villi, shown here, are small folds in the digestive system. Villi take nutrients from food and pass them to the blood.

This drawing shows red blood cells moving through a blood vessel.
Inset: Healthy red blood cells, such as the red ones in this picture, are round. The illness sickle-cell anemia changes the shape of red blood cells. The pink cells in this picture were changed by this illness.

What Is Blood?

As well as moving oxygen and waste to and from the cells, blood also helps the body stay warm. Blood carries heat made by the muscles and the organs throughout the body.

Blood is made up of cells suspended, or held, in a **liquid** called plasma. Plasma is made of water, oxygen, carbon dioxide, sugars, salts, and **proteins**. Most of the cells suspended in plasma are red blood cells. They look like flattened balls that bend in a bit on each side. Red blood cells carry oxygen to the body's cells.

White Blood Cells and Platelets

Along with red blood cells, plasma carries white blood cells and platelets. White blood cells help guard the body against harmful cells, such as **bacteria**. Harmful cells can enter organ tissue and blood. White blood cells discover and destroy the harmful cells.

Platelets help mend **wounds**. When tissue is cut, the blood spills out from the vessels that run through that tissue. Platelets build up at the wound. They work with a protein found in nearby tissue to form a web across the wound. The web slowly hardens and stops the blood loss.

In this picture a white blood cell, shown in blue, is folding around a harmful cell, shown in yellow. *Inset:* Red blood cells, white blood cells, and platelets work to close a wound.

Put your thumb on the artery in your wrist. You should feel a beat. This is called a pulse. It happens each time your heart pumps. *Inset:* Red blood cells move through a small artery.

Arteries are vessels that carry blood away from the heart. The largest artery, the aorta, carries oxygen-rich blood from the left ventricle to cells throughout the body. A smaller artery, called the pulmonary trunk, carries oxygen-poor blood from the right ventricle to the lungs. As the arteries move away from the heart, they branch out into smaller vessels. The smallest arteries are called capillaries. Plasma can move through the thin walls of the capillaries. This is how nutrients enter the tissues of organs and muscles.

Veins

Veins are vessels that carry blood toward the heart. Just as streams come together to form rivers, thin veins meet to form larger and larger vessels leading to the heart. The superior vena cava and the inferior vena cava are the largest of these vessels. Oxygen-poor blood from throughout the body travels through these veins to the heart's right atrium. From there the blood goes to the right ventricle and then to the lungs. The pulmonary veins bring oxygen-rich blood from the lungs to the left atrium of the heart.

This picture of the vena cava was taken by an x-ray. An x-ray is a machine that can take pictures inside the body. *Inset:* In some people's hands, the veins push up at the skin so you can see them.

21

Problems of the Heart

The most common circulatory problem is heart disease. Heart disease is the buildup of fatty matter called plaque in the arteries. Plaque slows the flow of blood. This causes angina, or great pain in the chest. Plaque can also cause a heart attack. A heart attack happens when one of the vessels that carries blood to the heart becomes blocked.

The way you live can help guard you from heart disease. Exercising and eating foods that are low in fat and rich in nutrients will help keep your circulatory system healthy.

Glossary

bacteria (bak-TEER-ee-uh) Tiny living things that cannot be seen with the eye alone. Some bacteria cause illness or rotting, but others are helpful.

blood vessels (BLUD VEH-suhlz) Narrow tunnels in the body, through which blood flows.

digestive system (dy-JES-tiv SIS-tem) The body parts that help turn the food you eat into the power your body needs.

harmful (HARM-ful) Causing hurt.

liquid (LIH-kwed) Matter that moves like water.

lungs (LUNGZ) The parts of an air-breathing animal that take in air and supply oxygen to the blood.

muscle (MUH-sul) A part of the body that is used to make the body move.

nutrients (NOO-tree-ints) Food that a living thing needs to live and grow.

organ (OR-gen) A part inside the body that does a job.

oxygen (OK-sih-jen) A gas that has no color or taste and is necessary for people and animals to breathe.

proteins (PROH-teenz) Important parts of the cells of all plants and animals.

respiratory system (RES-puh-ruh-tor-ee SIS-tem) The parts of the body that help in breathing.

tissue (TIH-shoo) Matter that forms the parts of living things.

wounds (WOONDZ) Places where the body is hurt and bleeding.

Index

A

arteries, 8, 19

C

capillaries, 8, 19
carbon dioxide, 4,
    11, 15
cells, 4, 11–12,
    15–16

D

digestive system, 4,
    12

H

heart, 4, 7–8, 11,
    19–20, 22

L

lungs, 7, 11,
    19–20

M

muscle(s), 7–8,
    15, 19

N

nutrients, 4, 12, 19

O

oxygen, 4, 11, 15,
    19–20

P

plasma, 15–16, 19
protein(s), 15–16

R

respiratory system,
    4, 11

V

veins, 8, 20

Web Sites

Due to the changing nature of Internet links, PowerKids Press has developed an online list of Web sites related to the subject of this book. This site is updated regularly. Please use this link to access the list: www.powerkidslinks.com/hybw/circulat/